Stretching Exercises For Seniors Over 50

A Comprehensive Guide to Effective Transformative Stretching Practices For Flexibility and Mobility For Active Aging

Juanita T. Williams

Table of Contents

CHAPTER ONE:

Introduction

Stretching is often undervalued and overlooked, especially among seniors. However, its importance cannot be overstated, particularly for older adults looking to maintain their mobility, flexibility, and overall quality of life.

In this introduction, we'll delve into the profound understanding of why stretching plays a pivotal role in the lives of older adults, explore the multitude of benefits it offers, and discuss essential safety precautions and guidelines to ensure a safe and effective stretching practice.

Understanding the Importance of Stretching for Seniors

As we age, our bodies undergo various changes, including a natural decline in muscle mass, flexibility, and joint mobility. Without proper attention and care, these changes can lead to stiffness, decreased range of motion, and an increased risk of injury. This is where stretching comes in as a vital component of a senior's fitness routine.

Stretching helps counteract the effects of aging on the musculoskeletal system by promoting flexibility and joint mobility. It lengthens muscles and tendons, which can alleviate tension and improve overall movement patterns.

For seniors, maintaining or improving flexibility is essential for performing daily activities with ease, such as bending down to tie shoelaces, reaching for items on high shelves, or getting in and out of chairs.

Moreover, regular stretching can enhance balance and coordination, reducing the risk of falls—a significant concern among older adults. By improving proprioception (the body's awareness of its position in space) and enhancing muscle control, seniors can feel more confident in their movements and reduce the likelihood of accidents that could result in injury or loss of independence.

In addition to physical benefits, stretching also offers mental and emotional advantages for seniors. It provides an opportunity for relaxation and stress relief, promoting a sense of well-being and overall mental clarity.

Benefits of Stretching for Older Adults

Here are some of the key advantages seniors can experience by incorporating regular stretching into their lives:

1. **Improved Range of Motion**: Stretching helps seniors maintain or regain their ability to move joints through their full range of motion, allowing for greater freedom of movement in daily activities.

2. **Enhanced Flexibility**: Increased flexibility can alleviate stiffness and discomfort, making it easier for seniors to perform tasks that require bending, reaching, or twisting.

3. **Prevention of Injury and Falls**: Maintaining flexibility and joint mobility is paramount for reducing the risk of falls and injuries, which can have devastating consequences for seniors. By regularly stretching major muscle groups and improving proprioception, seniors can enhance their body awareness and

coordination, mitigating the likelihood of accidents.

4. **Enhanced Posture and Alignment**: Poor posture is a common consequence of aging, exacerbated by sedentary lifestyles and muscular imbalances. Stretching targets key muscle groups responsible for maintaining proper posture, such as the chest, shoulders, and hip flexors, helping seniors stand taller and straighter with greater ease and comfort.

5. **Stress Relief**: Engaging in stretching can promote relaxation and reduce tension in both the body and mind, providing seniors with a natural way to manage stress and promote overall well-being.

6. **Improved Circulation**: Stretching increases blood flow to muscles and tissues, which can help seniors maintain healthy circulation and prevent issues such as swelling or numbness in the extremities.

7. **Enhanced Athletic Performance**: For seniors who participate in sports or

recreational activities, stretching can improve performance by increasing flexibility, agility, and balance.

8. **Enhanced Muscle Strength and Function**: Contrary to popular belief, stretching is not solely about lengthening muscles; it also plays a crucial role in strengthening them. By elongating muscle fibers and improving their alignment, stretching exercises promote optimal muscle function and performance, thereby enhancing stability and balance.

9. **Alleviation of Chronic Pain**: Chronic pain is a pervasive issue among older adults, often stemming from musculoskeletal imbalances and inflammatory conditions. Stretching offers a natural and non-invasive approach to pain management, relieving tension in tight muscles and promoting relaxation in overactive ones. Additionally, stretching exercises stimulate the release of endorphins, the body's natural painkillers, providing relief from discomfort and improving overall quality of life.

Safety Precautions and Guidelines

Here, we outline essential safety precautions and guidelines to help seniors embark on their stretching journey with confidence and peace of mind:

1. **Consult with a healthcare professional**: Before initiating any new exercise regimen, seniors should consult with their healthcare provider to assess their individual fitness level and identify any underlying medical conditions or contraindications that may impact their ability to stretch safely.

2. **Start slowly and progress gradually**: Rome wasn't built in a day, and neither should one's flexibility. Begin with gentle stretching exercises, focusing on major muscle groups and joints, and gradually increase the intensity and duration of their stretches as their flexibility improves. Avoid pushing past your comfort level or bouncing in stretches, as this can increase the risk of injury.

3. **Listen to your body**: Pain is not synonymous with progress. Seniors should pay close attention to their bodies'

signals during stretching exercises and avoid pushing themselves beyond their limits. Discomfort may be normal, but sharp or shooting pain is a sign of potential injury and should be heeded accordingly.

4. **Warm-up before stretching**: Cold muscles are more prone to injury, so it's essential for seniors to warm up their bodies before engaging in stretching activities. A brief cardiovascular warm-up, such as brisk walking or gentle cycling, can help increase blood flow to the muscles and prepare them for stretching.

5. **Use Proper Technique:** Form and alignment are paramount in stretching to ensure efficacy and safety. Seniors should perform each stretch with precision and control, avoiding bouncing or jerking movements that can strain the muscles and ligaments. It may be helpful to seek guidance from a qualified fitness professional or physical therapist to learn proper stretching techniques.

6. **Hold stretches for an appropriate duration**: Aim to hold each stretch for

15-30 seconds, breathing deeply and gradually increasing the stretch if comfortable. Avoid holding your breath or overstretching.

7. **Incorporate variety:** Include a variety of stretching techniques, such as static, dynamic, and proprioceptive neuromuscular facilitation (PNF) stretches, to target different muscle groups and improve overall flexibility.

8. **Stay Hydrated and Well-Nourished**: Hydration and nutrition play a vital role in supporting overall health and recovery. Seniors should ensure they are adequately hydrated before and after stretching exercises and consume a balanced diet rich in nutrients to fuel their bodies and promote tissue repair and regeneration.

CHAPTER TWO:

Getting Started with Stretching

In this section, we guide you through the crucial steps of getting started with stretching, from assessing your current flexibility and mobility to setting realistic goals and establishing a consistent routine.

Assessing Your Current Flexibility and Mobility

Consider the following steps to conduct a self-assessment:

1. **Range of Motion Checks**: Begin by gently moving each joint through its full range of motion. Take note of any areas where movement feels restricted or uncomfortable. This can help identify specific areas that may require additional attention during your stretching routine.

2. **Muscle Flexibility**: Perform basic stretches for major muscle groups, such as the hamstrings, quadriceps, shoulders,

and back. Pay attention to how easily you can move into each stretch and whether there is tightness or discomfort. This provides insights into your muscle flexibility and areas that may benefit from targeted stretching.

3. **Postural Analysis**: Observe your standing and sitting posture. Note any imbalances or areas of tension, such as rounded shoulders or a forward head position. These observations will guide you in selecting stretches that address specific postural issues.

4. **Joint Mobility**: Assess the mobility of key joints, including ankles, knees, hips, and shoulders. Gentle joint mobilization exercises can help improve joint fluidity and identify areas where increased mobility is needed.

Setting Realistic Goals

Consider the following principles when establishing your stretching goals:

1. **Specificity**: Clearly define your stretching goals, focusing on specific areas or muscle groups you wish to improve.

Whether it's increasing hamstring flexibility, improving shoulder mobility, or addressing overall posture, specificity enhances the effectiveness of your stretching routine.

2. **Measurable Targets**: Set measurable benchmarks to track your progress. This could involve tracking the distance you can comfortably reach in a particular stretch, the duration of a stretch, or the improvement in your overall range of motion. Measurable targets provide tangible evidence of your achievements.

3. **Realistic Expectations**: Be realistic about the time frame and magnitude of your goals. Rome wasn't built in a day, and significant improvements in flexibility may take time. Setting achievable milestones prevents frustration and encourages a positive mindset.

4. **Adaptability**: Recognize that goals may need to be adjusted based on your body's response to stretching. Listen to your body, and be open to modifying your goals if necessary. Adaptability ensures

that your stretching routine remains a sustainable and enjoyable part of your lifestyle.

5. **Long-Term Vision**: Consider both short-term and long-term goals. While immediate improvements are gratifying, envisioning the long-term benefits of a consistent stretching practice reinforces its role as a lifelong commitment to health and well-being.

Creating a Consistent Routine

Here's how to establish a consistent stretching routine:

1. **Set a Schedule**: Designate specific times for your stretching sessions. Whether it's in the morning to kickstart your day or in the evening to unwind, having a set schedule helps integrate stretching into your daily routine.

2. **Start Small:** Begin with a manageable duration for your stretching routine. A 10-15 minute session can be highly effective and is more likely to be maintained consistently than a longer, more time-intensive routine.

3. **Incorporate Variety**: Keep your routine interesting by incorporating a variety of stretches that target different muscle groups and areas of the body. This prevents monotony and ensures a comprehensive approach to flexibility.

4. **Use Reminders**: Set reminders or alarms on your phone to prompt your stretching sessions. Consistent reminders can help overcome resistance and establish a routine over time.

5. **Combine with Other Activities**: Integrate stretching into your existing activities. For example, stretch while watching TV, waiting for the kettle to boil, or during work breaks. This makes stretching a seamless part of your daily life.

6. **Progress Gradually**: As your flexibility improves, gradually progress your routine by adding new stretches or increasing the duration of existing ones. This incremental approach prevents overwhelm and supports continual growth.

CHAPTER THREE:

Warm-Up Exercises

In this section, we explore three essential components of a comprehensive warm-up routine: gentle cardiovascular warm-up, joint mobilization exercises, and dynamic stretching for increased blood flow.

Gentle Cardiovascular Warm-Up

Consider the following guidelines for incorporating a cardiovascular warm-up into your stretching routine:

1. **Duration**: Aim for a cardiovascular warm-up lasting 5-10 minutes, gradually increasing the intensity as your body adjusts to the activity.

2. **Intensity**: Keep the intensity of your warm-up moderate, focusing on maintaining a steady pace that elevates your heart rate without causing fatigue or breathlessness.

3. **Range of Motion**: Incorporate movements that engage multiple muscle

groups and joints, such as arm circles, leg swings, and torso twists, to promote full-body mobilization and preparation for stretching.

4. **Variety**: Keep your warm-up routine varied and enjoyable by alternating between different activities, such as brisk walking, marching, or cycling on a stationary bike. This prevents boredom and ensures a well-rounded warm-up experience.

5. **Gradual Progression**: As your fitness level improves, gradually increase the intensity and duration of your cardiovascular warm-up to continue challenging your body and maximizing its readiness for stretching.

Joint Mobilization Exercises

Consider the following joint mobilization exercises to incorporate into your warm-up routine:

1. **Neck Circles**: Slowly rotate your head in a circular motion, moving from side to side and front to back to mobilize the

cervical spine and relieve tension in the neck and shoulders.

2. **Shoulder Rolls**: Roll your shoulders in a circular motion, moving them forward and backward to improve mobility and circulation in the shoulder joints.

3. **Wrist Circles**: Rotate your wrists in a circular motion, moving them clockwise and counterclockwise to increase flexibility and relieve stiffness in the wrists and forearms.

4. **Hip Circles**: Stand with feet hip-width apart and gently rotate your hips in a circular motion, moving them clockwise and counterclockwise to improve mobility and reduce tightness in the hip joints.

5. **Ankle Alphabet**: Sit or stand with one foot lifted off the ground and trace the letters of the alphabet with your big toe, moving your ankle through its full range of motion to improve mobility and proprioception.

Dynamic Stretching for Increased Blood Flow

Dynamic stretching involves moving the body through a range of motion in a controlled and fluid manner, actively engaging the muscles and promoting increased blood flow to the tissues.

Unlike static stretching, which involves holding a stretch for an extended period, dynamic stretching focuses on movement and rhythm, preparing the muscles for the demands of physical activity.

Consider the following dynamic stretching exercises to incorporate into your warm-up routine:

1. **Leg Swings**: Stand facing a wall or support and swing one leg forward and backward in a controlled motion, gradually increasing the range of motion with each swing to stretch the hamstrings and hip flexors.

2. **Arm Circles**: Extend your arms out to the sides and make circular motions with your arms, gradually increasing the size of

the circles to warm up the shoulder joints and upper body muscles.

3. **Torso Twists**: Stand with feet shoulder-width apart and rotate your torso from side to side, allowing your arms to swing freely to stretch the spine and engage the core muscles.

4. **Walking Lunges**: Take a step forward with one foot and lower your body into a lunge position, keeping your front knee aligned with your ankle. Push off the front foot to return to the starting position and repeat on the other side to dynamically stretch the hip flexors, quadriceps, and glutes.

5. **Leg Kicks**: Stand with feet hip-width apart and kick one leg forward, aiming to touch your toes with your hand while keeping the leg straight. Alternate legs in a dynamic motion to stretch the hamstrings and improve flexibility in the legs.

CHAPTER FOUR:

Upper Body Stretching

The upper body, comprising the neck, shoulders, chest, arms, and wrists, is a focal point for tension and tightness, particularly in individuals who spend prolonged periods sitting or engaging in repetitive movements.

In this section, we explore three essential components of an effective upper body stretching routine: neck and shoulder stretches, chest opener exercises, and arm and wrist stretches.

Neck and Shoulder Stretches

The neck and shoulders bear the brunt of modern-day stressors, including prolonged sitting, computer use, and poor posture, often resulting in stiffness, tension, and discomfort. Consider the following neck and shoulder stretches to include in your routine:

1. **Neck Side Stretch**: Sit or stand tall and gently tilt your head to one side, bringing your ear towards your shoulder until you feel a stretch along the side of your neck.

Repeat on the other side after holding for 15–30 seconds.

2. **Neck Rotation**: Turn your head to one side, bringing your chin towards your shoulder, and hold for 15-30 seconds. Repeat on the opposite side to stretch the muscles in the back of the neck.

3. **Shoulder Roll:** Shrug your shoulders up towards your ears, then roll them back in a circular motion, squeezing your shoulder blades together at the back. Repeat for 10-15 repetitions to release tension in the shoulders and upper back.

4. **Eagle Arms**: Extend your arms out to the sides, then cross one arm over the other at the elbows, wrapping the forearms and palms together. Lift your elbows slightly to feel a stretch in the upper back and shoulders. Switch sides after holding for 15 to 30 seconds.

5. **Upper Trapezius Stretch**: Sit or stand tall and gently tilt your head to one side, then use your hand to apply gentle pressure to the opposite side of your head, increasing the stretch along the side of

your neck and upper trapezius muscle. After holding for 15 to 30 seconds, switch to the other side.

Chest Opener Exercises

In today's sedentary lifestyle, prolonged sitting and hunching over electronic devices contribute to tightness and weakness in the chest muscles, leading to rounded shoulders and poor posture.

Chest opener exercises are designed to counteract these effects by stretching the chest muscles and opening up the front of the body. Consider the following chest opener exercises to include in your routine:

1. **Doorway Stretch**: Stand in a doorway with your arms extended out to the sides at shoulder height, palms resting against the door frame. Lean forward slightly to feel a stretch across the chest and front of the shoulders. Hold for 15-30 seconds, then release.

2. **Chest Expansion**: Sit or stand tall with your arms extended behind your back, clasping your hands together and pressing your palms towards each other. Lift your chest and draw your shoulder blades

together to deepen the stretch across the chest. Hold for 15-30 seconds, then release.

3. **Wall Stretch**: Stand facing a wall and place one hand against it at shoulder height, with your elbow slightly bent. Gently rotate your body away from the wall to feel a stretch across the chest and front of the shoulders. After holding for 15 to 30 seconds, swap sides.

4. **Pectoral Stretch**: Lie on your stomach with your arms extended out to the sides at shoulder height, palms facing down. Press into the ground with your hands and lift your chest, drawing your shoulder blades together to feel a stretch across the chest. Hold for 15-30 seconds, then release.

5. **Resistance Band Chest Stretch**: Hold a resistance band behind your back with your arms extended out to the sides at shoulder height. Gently pull the band apart to feel a stretch across the chest and front of the shoulders. Hold for 15-30 seconds, then release.

Arm and Wrist Stretches

The arms and wrists are often neglected in stretching routines, yet they play a crucial role in everyday activities and can benefit greatly from targeted stretches to alleviate tension and improve flexibility.

Consider the following arm and wrist stretches to include in your routine:

1. **Wrist Flexor Stretch**: Extend one arm out in front of you with the palm facing down. Use your other hand to gently press the fingers of the extended hand towards you until you feel a stretch in the wrist and forearm. After 15 to 30 seconds of holding, switch sides.

2. **Wrist Extensor Stretch**: Extend one arm out in front of you with the palm facing up. Use your other hand to gently press the fingers of the extended hand towards the floor until you feel a stretch in the wrist and back of the forearm. After 15 to 30 seconds of holding, switch sides.

3. **Triceps Stretch**: Reach one arm overhead and bend the elbow, placing your hand on the upper back between the

shoulder blades. Use your other hand to gently press the elbow towards the center of your head until you feel a stretch in the back of the arm. After 15 to 30 seconds of holding, switch sides.

4. **Biceps Stretch**: Extend one arm out in front of you with the palm facing up. Use your other hand to gently pull the fingers of the extended hand down towards the floor until you feel a stretch in the front of the arm. After 15 to 30 seconds of holding, switch sides.

5. **Forearm Stretch**: Extend one arm out in front of you with the palm facing down. Use your other hand to gently press the fingers of the extended hand towards the floor until you feel a stretch in the forearm. After 15 to 30 seconds of holding, switch sides.

CHAPTER FIVE:

Lower Body Stretching

The lower body bears the weight of daily activities and is often subjected to tightness and discomfort, particularly in individuals who lead sedentary lifestyles or engage in repetitive movements.

In this section, we explore three essential components of an effective lower body stretching routine: hip flexor and quadriceps stretches, hamstring and calf stretches, and ankle mobility exercises.

Hip Flexor and Quadriceps Stretches

The hip flexors and quadriceps are key muscle groups involved in walking, running, and maintaining proper posture. Prolonged sitting and inactivity can lead to tightness in these muscles, contributing to discomfort and restricted mobility.

Consider the following stretches to include in your routine:

1. **Kneeling Hip Flexor Stretch**: Kneel on one knee with the other foot planted flat on the floor in front of you. Engage your core and gently lean forward, pressing your hips towards the ground until you feel a stretch in the front of the hip and thigh of the kneeling leg. After 15 to 30 seconds of holding, switch sides.

2. **Standing Quadriceps Stretch**: Stand tall with feet hip-width apart. Bend one knee and bring your heel towards your buttocks, grasping your ankle with your hand. Keep your knees together and gently press your hips forward until you feel a stretch in the front of the thigh. After 15 to 30 seconds of holding, switch sides.

3. **Lunging Hip Flexor Stretch**: Step one foot forward into a lunge position, bending the front knee and keeping the back leg straight. Engage your core and gently shift your weight forward, pressing your hips towards the ground until you feel a stretch in the front of the hip and thigh of the back leg. After 15 to 30 seconds of holding, switch sides.

4. **Seated Quadriceps Stretch**: Sit on the ground with your legs extended in front of you. Bend one knee and bring your heel towards your buttocks, placing your foot flat on the ground. Gently lean back onto your hands and lift your chest, pressing your hips forward until you feel a stretch in the front of the thigh. After 15 to 30 seconds of holding, switch sides.

5. **Pigeon Pose:** Begin in a tabletop position with your hands and knees on the ground. Bring one knee forward and place it behind your wrist, with your shin angled across your body. Extend your opposite leg straight back behind you. Lower your hips towards the ground, feeling a stretch in the front of the hip and thigh of the extended leg. After 15 to 30 seconds of holding, switch sides.

Hamstring and Calf Stretches

The hamstrings and calves are integral to lower body movement and are often prone to tightness and stiffness, particularly in individuals who engage in activities such as running or cycling.

Consider the following stretches to include in your routine:

1. **Standing Hamstring Stretch**: Stand tall with feet hip-width apart. Extend one leg forward and place your heel on a raised surface, such as a step or bench. Keep your knee straight and hinge forward at the hips, reaching towards your toes until you feel a stretch in the back of the thigh. After 15 to 30 seconds of holding, switch sides.

2. **Seated Hamstring Stretch**: Sit on the ground with your legs extended in front of you. Bend one knee and place the sole of your foot against the inner thigh of the opposite leg. Hinge forward at the hips, reaching towards your toes until you feel a stretch in the back of the extended leg. After 15 to 30 seconds of holding, switch sides.

3. **Calf Stretch Against Wall**: Stand facing a wall with your hands resting against it at shoulder height. Step one foot back and press your heel into the ground, keeping your back leg straight and your knee bent. Feel the back leg's calf stretch as you slant forward a little. After 15 to 30 seconds of holding, switch sides.

4. **Downward Dog Pose**: Begin in a tabletop position with your hands and knees on the ground. Lift your hips towards the ceiling, straightening your arms and legs to form an inverted V shape with your body. Press your heels towards the ground, feeling a stretch in the calves and hamstrings. Hold for 15-30 seconds, then release.

5. **Seated Calf Stretch**: Sit on the ground with your legs extended in front of you. Loop a resistance band around the ball of one foot and hold onto the ends with your hands. Flex your foot and gently pull the resistance band towards you until you feel a stretch in the calf. After holding for 15 to 30 seconds, swap sides.

Ankle Mobility Exercises

The ankles play a crucial role in balance, stability, and mobility, yet they are often neglected in stretching routines. Poor ankle mobility can lead to compensatory movements and increased risk of injury in the lower body.

Consider the following ankle mobility exercises to include in your routine:

1. **Ankle Circles**: Sit or stand with your feet flat on the ground. Lift one foot off the ground and gently rotate your ankle in a circular motion, moving clockwise and counterclockwise to improve mobility in all directions. After ten to fifteen repetitions, swap sides.

2. **Toe Taps**: Sit or stand with your feet flat on the ground. Lift one foot off the ground and tap your toes on the floor in front of you, then return to the starting position. After ten to fifteen repetitions, swap sides.

3. **Heel Raises**: Stand tall with feet hip-width apart. Lift your heels off the ground and rise up onto the balls of your feet, then lower back down to the starting position. Repeat for 10-15 repetitions to strengthen the muscles around the ankles and improve mobility.

4. **Ankle Dorsiflexion Stretch**: Sit on the ground with your legs extended in front of you. Loop a resistance band around the ball of one foot and hold onto the ends with your hands. Flex your foot and gently pull the resistance band towards you until

you feel a stretch in the front of the ankle. After holding for 15 to 30 seconds, swap sides.

5. **Calf Raises**: Stand tall with feet hip-width apart. Rise up onto the balls of your feet, lifting your heels off the ground as high as you can. Hold for a moment at the top, then lower back down to the starting position. Repeat for 10-15 repetitions to strengthen the muscles around the ankles and improve mobility.

CHAPTER SIX:

Core and Back Stretches

The core and back muscles play a fundamental role in maintaining stability, posture, and overall body function. In this section, we explore three essential components of an effective core and back stretching routine: spinal rotation stretches, abdominal strengthening and stretching, and lower back release techniques.

Spinal Rotation Stretches

Spinal rotation stretches are designed to improve flexibility and mobility in the spine, promoting healthy movement patterns and reducing the risk of discomfort and injury. Consider the following spinal rotation stretches to include in your routine:

1. **Seated Spinal Twist**: Sit on the ground with your legs extended in front of you. Bend one knee and cross it over the opposite leg, placing the foot flat on the ground. Place the opposite hand on the outside of the bent knee and gently twist towards the bent leg, placing the other

hand behind you for support. After holding for 15 to 30 seconds, swap sides.

2. **Supine Spinal Twist**: Lie on your back with your arms extended out to the sides at shoulder height. Bend your knees and lift them towards your chest, then lower them to one side, allowing your hips to rotate towards the ground. Keep your shoulders flat on the ground and gaze towards the opposite hand. After holding for 15 to 30 seconds, swap sides..

3. **Standing Spinal Twist**: Stand tall with feet hip-width apart. Raise your arms shoulder-high and out to the sides. Gently rotate your torso to one side, keeping your hips facing forward and your feet firmly planted on the ground. After holding for 15 to 30 seconds, swap sides.

4. **Seated Cat-Cow Stretch**: Sit on the ground with your legs crossed in front of you. Place your hands on your knees and arch your back, lifting your chest towards the ceiling and gazing upwards (Cow Pose). Then, round your spine and tuck your chin towards your chest, drawing your belly button towards your spine (Cat

Pose). Repeat for 5-10 repetitions to gently mobilize the spine.

5. **Standing Trunk Rotation:** Stand tall with feet hip-width apart and hands on your hips. Slowly rotate your torso to one side, keeping your hips facing forward and your feet planted on the ground. Hold for 15-30 seconds, then return to the starting position and repeat on the opposite side.

Abdominal Strengthening and Stretching

The abdominal muscles, often referred to as the "core," are essential for maintaining stability, supporting proper posture, and protecting the spine. Consider the following abdominal strengthening and stretching exercises to include in your routine:

1. **Plank Pose**: Begin in a push-up position with your hands shoulder-width apart and your body in a straight line from head to heels. Engage your core and hold this position for 30-60 seconds, focusing on maintaining proper alignment and breathing deeply.

2. **Supine Leg Raises**: Lie on your back with your legs extended straight and your arms at your sides. Engage your core and lift both legs towards the ceiling, keeping them straight and together. Lower them back down towards the ground, hovering just above the floor, then lift them back up. Repeat for 10-15 repetitions.

3. **Seated Forward Fold:** Sit on the ground with your legs extended in front of you. Engage your core and hinge forward at the hips, reaching towards your toes with your hands. Keep your back straight and your chest lifted, feeling a stretch in the hamstrings and lower back. Hold for 15-30 seconds, then release.

4. **Bridge Pose**: Lie on your back with your knees bent and feet flat on the ground hip-width apart. Press into your feet and lift your hips towards the ceiling, engaging your glutes and core. Hold this position for 15-30 seconds, then lower back down to the ground.

5. **Standing Side Stretch**: Stand tall with feet hip-width apart and arms extended

overhead. Gently lean to one side, reaching towards the sky with your fingertips and feeling a stretch along the side of your body. Hold for 15-30 seconds, then return to the starting position and repeat on the opposite side.

Lower Back Release Techniques

The lower back, or lumbar spine, is a common site of discomfort and tension, particularly in individuals who spend prolonged periods sitting or engaging in activities that place stress on the spine. Consider the following lower back release techniques to include in your routine:

1. **Supine Knee-to-Chest Stretch**: Lie on your back with your knees bent and feet flat on the ground. Bring one knee towards your chest and clasp your hands around it, gently pulling it towards you until you feel a stretch in the lower back. After holding for 15 to 30 seconds, switch sides.

2. **Child's Pose:** Begin on your hands and knees with your toes touching and knees apart. Sit back onto your heels and extend your arms forward, lowering your chest towards the ground and resting your

forehead on the mat. Feel a stretch in your lower back and hips. Hold for 30-60 seconds, breathing deeply.

3. **Seated Forward Bend**: Sit on the ground with your legs extended in front of you. Engage your core and hinge forward at the hips, reaching towards your toes with your hands. Keep your back straight and your chest lifted, feeling a stretch in the hamstrings and lower back. Hold for 15-30 seconds, then release.

4. **Cat-Cow Stretch:** Begin on your hands and knees with your wrists directly under your shoulders and your knees under your hips. Inhale as you arch your back, lifting your chest and tailbone towards the ceiling (Cow Pose). Exhale as you round your back, tucking your chin towards your chest and pressing into the ground with your hands (Cat Pose). Repeat for 5-10 repetitions, flowing smoothly between the two poses.

5. **Seated Spinal Twist:** Sit on the ground with your legs extended in front of you. Bend one knee and cross

it over the opposite leg, placing the foot flat on the ground. Place the opposite hand on the outside of the bent knee and gently twist towards the bent leg, placing the other hand behind you for support. After holding for 15 to 30 seconds, switch sides.

CHAPTER SEVEN:

Flexibility Challenges for Seniors

Flexibility is a cornerstone of healthy aging, yet many seniors face unique challenges when it comes to maintaining or improving their flexibility. Factors such as age-related changes in the musculoskeletal system, previous injuries, and medical conditions can present obstacles to achieving optimal flexibility.

In this section, we explore three common challenges faced by seniors when it comes to flexibility: overcoming common obstacles, modifying stretches for individual needs, and dealing with arthritis and joint pain.

Overcoming Common Obstacles

As we age, the body undergoes natural changes that can affect flexibility, including loss of muscle mass, decreased joint mobility, and changes in connective tissue elasticity. Additionally, seniors may face lifestyle factors such as sedentary behavior or chronic health conditions that further impact flexibility.

Consider the following strategies to overcome common flexibility challenges:

1. **Gradual Progression**: Start slowly and gradually increase the intensity and duration of your stretching routine over time. Focus on gentle, controlled movements and listen to your body's feedback to avoid overexertion or injury.

2. **Consistency**: Establishing a consistent stretching routine is key to improving flexibility. Set aside time each day for stretching exercises, and make it a priority to stick to your routine even on days when you may not feel like it.

3. **Variety**: Incorporate a variety of stretching exercises into your routine to target different muscle groups and movement patterns. This helps prevent boredom and ensures that you are addressing all areas of your body that may be tight or stiff.

4. **Use of Props:** Consider using props such as yoga blocks, straps, or bolsters to support your body in certain stretches and

make them more accessible. Props can help modify stretches to accommodate limited flexibility or mobility.

5. **Mindfulness**: Approach your stretching routine with mindfulness and awareness, paying attention to your breath, body sensations, and any areas of tension or discomfort. Mindful stretching can help improve body awareness and enhance the effectiveness of your practice.

Modifying Stretches for Individual Needs

Seniors come from diverse backgrounds and may have varying levels of flexibility, mobility, and strength. As such, it's important to modify stretches to meet individual needs and abilities. Consider the following tips for modifying stretches for individual needs:

1. **Range of Motion**: Adapt stretches to accommodate limited range of motion by reducing the intensity or amplitude of the movement. Focus on moving within a comfortable range and gradually increasing flexibility over time.

2. **Supportive Equipment**: Use supportive equipment such as chairs, walls, or cushions to assist with balance and stability during stretches. This can help seniors maintain proper alignment and reduce the risk of falls or injury.

3. **Seated Stretches**: Many stretches can be modified to be performed while seated in a chair or wheelchair. Seated stretches are ideal for seniors with mobility limitations or those who may have difficulty getting down on the floor.

4. **Gentle Progression**: Start with gentle, basic stretches and gradually progress to more advanced variations as flexibility improves. Encourage seniors to listen to their bodies and avoid pushing themselves too hard, especially if they are new to stretching or have underlying health conditions.

5. **Individualized Approach**: Work with a qualified fitness professional or physical therapist to develop a personalized stretching program tailored to your individual needs, goals, and medical history. A customized approach ensures

that stretches are safe, effective, and appropriate for your unique circumstances.

Dealing with Arthritis and Joint Pain

Arthritis and joint pain are common concerns for seniors and can significantly impact flexibility and mobility. Arthritis, in particular, can cause inflammation, stiffness, and pain in the joints, making it challenging to engage in regular stretching activities.

Consider the following strategies for dealing with arthritis and joint pain:

1. **Low-Impact Exercises:** Choose low-impact exercises such as swimming, cycling, or tai chi that are gentle on the joints and promote flexibility without exacerbating arthritis symptoms. These activities help improve range of motion, reduce stiffness, and alleviate joint pain.

2. **Warm-Up:** Prior to stretching, engage in a gentle cardiovascular warm-up to increase blood flow to the muscles and joints, preparing them for stretching

activities. A warm-up helps reduce stiffness and improves flexibility, making stretches more effective.

3. **Joint Protection**: When performing stretches, use proper technique and avoid overexerting or forcing joints beyond their comfortable range of motion. Focus on gentle, controlled movements and listen to your body's feedback to avoid aggravating arthritis symptoms.

4. **Range-of-Motion Exercises**: Incorporate range-of-motion exercises that specifically target the affected joints, such as gentle wrist circles, shoulder rolls, or ankle rotations. These exercises help lubricate the joints, reduce stiffness, and improve flexibility.

5. **Pain Management**: Use pain management techniques such as heat therapy, cold therapy, or over-the-counter pain relievers to alleviate arthritis symptoms and reduce discomfort during stretching activities. For individualized advice, speak with a medical expert.

CHAPTER EIGHT:

Cool-Down and Relaxation Techniques

As essential as it is to engage in physical activity and stretching exercises, it is equally important to allow the body to cool down and relax afterward. Cool-down and relaxation techniques not only help prevent injury and muscle soreness but also promote mental and emotional well-being.

In this section, we explore three effective techniques for cooling down and relaxing the body and mind: deep breathing exercises, mindfulness and meditation practices, and incorporating foam rolling and self-massage.

Deep Breathing Exercises

Deep breathing exercises are a simple yet powerful way to calm the mind, reduce stress, and promote relaxation. Consider the following deep breathing exercises to include in your cool-down routine:

1. **Diaphragmatic Breathing**: Sit or lie down in a comfortable position with your eyes closed. Put your hands on your chest and your abdomen, respectively. Breathe deeply through your nose, letting your abdomen grow larger as air fills your lungs. Exhale slowly and completely through your mouth, feeling your abdomen deflate. Repeat for several breaths, focusing on the sensation of deep, rhythmic breathing.

2. **4-7-8 Breathing**: Sit or lie down in a comfortable position and close your eyes. Inhale deeply through your nose for a count of 4 seconds, allowing your abdomen to expand. Take a deep breath and hold it for seven seconds. Exhale slowly and completely through your mouth for a count of 8 seconds, emptying your lungs. Repeat for several cycles, focusing on the length and rhythm of your breath.

3. **Alternate Nostril Breathing**: Sit in a comfortable position with your spine straight and your eyes closed. Your left hand should be palm up on your left knee. Use your right hand to place your index

and middle fingers between your eyebrows. Breathe deeply through your left nostril while closing your right nostril with your thumb. With your ring finger closed, open your left nostril, let go of your right, and exhale slowly and thoroughly. Inhale deeply through your right nostril, then close it with your right thumb and exhale through your left nostril. Repeat for several cycles, alternating nostrils with each breath.

4. **Counted Breathing**: Sit or lie down in a comfortable position and close your eyes. Inhale deeply through your nose for a count of 4 seconds. For four seconds, hold your breath. Exhale slowly and completely through your mouth for a count of 6 seconds. Hold your breath out for a count of 2 seconds. Repeat for several cycles, focusing on the rhythm of your breath and the sensation of relaxation.

Mindfulness and Meditation Practices

Mindfulness and meditation practices offer a powerful way to cultivate presence, awareness, and inner peace. Consider the following mindfulness and meditation practices to include in your cool-down routine:

1. **Body Scan Meditation**: Lie down in a comfortable position with your eyes closed. Start at your toes and slowly work your way up through your body, bringing awareness to each body part and noticing any sensations or tension. Take deep breaths and consciously relax each muscle group as you scan through your body. Continue until you reach the top of your head, feeling a sense of relaxation and openness throughout your body.

2. **Guided Visualization**: Sit or lie down in a comfortable position and close your eyes. Imagine yourself in a peaceful, serene setting such as a beach, forest, or mountaintop. Use your senses to immerse yourself in the scene, noticing the sights, sounds, smells, and sensations around you. Allow yourself to fully experience the relaxation and tranquility of the visualization, letting go of any stress or tension.

3. **Breath Awareness Meditation**: Sit in a comfortable position with your spine

straight and your eyes closed. Bring your attention to your breath, noticing the sensation of air entering and leaving your nostrils. Focus on the rise and fall of your chest and abdomen with each inhale and exhale. Remind yourself to breathe slowly and without passing judgment if your thoughts stray. Continue for several minutes, allowing yourself to sink deeper into a state of relaxation and presence.

4. **Loving-Kindness Meditation:** Sit or lie down in a comfortable position and close your eyes. Bring to mind someone you care about deeply, such as a friend, family member, or loved one. Repeat silently to yourself, "May you be happy, may you be healthy, may you be safe, may you be at ease." Extend these wishes to yourself, then gradually to others in your life, and finally to all beings everywhere. Feel a sense of warmth, compassion, and connection as you cultivate loving-kindness towards yourself and others.

Incorporating Foam Rolling and Self-Massage

Foam rolling and self-massage are effective techniques for relieving muscle tension, improving flexibility, and promoting relaxation. Consider the following techniques for incorporating foam rolling and self-massage into your cool-down routine:

1. **Foam Rolling for the Back:** Lie down on a foam roller with it positioned horizontally beneath your upper back. Support your head with your hands and gently roll back and forth along the length of your spine, focusing on areas of tightness or discomfort. Use your legs to control the pressure and intensity of the massage. Continue for several minutes, breathing deeply and allowing your muscles to relax and release tension.

2. **Massage Ball for the Feet**: Sit in a chair and place a massage ball or tennis ball beneath one foot. Roll the ball back and forth along the length of your foot, applying pressure to areas of tension or discomfort. Use your hands to control the intensity of the massage and focus on

areas such as the arches, heels, and balls of the feet. Continue for several minutes, then switch to the other foot.

3. **Foam Rolling for the Legs**: Sit on the floor with a foam roller positioned beneath one thigh. Place your hands on the ground behind you for support and use your arms to lift your hips off the ground. Roll back and forth along the length of your thigh, focusing on areas of tightness or discomfort. Use your hands and legs to control the pressure and intensity of the massage. Continue for several minutes, then switch to the other thigh.

4. **Self-Massage for the Shoulders**: Stand tall with a massage ball or tennis ball against a wall. Place the ball between your shoulder blade and the wall, then lean into the ball to apply pressure to the muscles of the upper back and shoulders. Move the ball around to target different areas of tension or discomfort. Use your body weight to control the intensity of the massage. Go to the opposite side after a few minutes of this.

CHAPTER NINE:

Stretching for Specific Health Conditions

While stretching offers numerous benefits for individuals of all ages and fitness levels, it can be especially beneficial for those with specific health conditions. Stretching exercises can help alleviate symptoms, improve function, and enhance overall well-being in individuals managing various health concerns.

In this section, we explore three common health conditions—osteoporosis and bone health, diabetes and blood circulation, and chronic pain—and how stretching can play a valuable role in managing these conditions.

Osteoporosis and Bone Health

Weakening of the bones, which increases their vulnerability to fractures and breaks, is the hallmark of osteoporosis. It is particularly prevalent among older adults, especially postmenopausal women, due to age-related bone loss.

Consider the following stretching exercises tailored for individuals with osteoporosis:

1. **Gentle Spine Stretch:** Sit tall in a chair with your feet flat on the ground and your hands resting on your thighs. Slowly rotate your torso to one side, placing one hand on the back of the chair for support and the other hand on your opposite knee. Hold the stretch for 15-30 seconds, then return to the starting position and repeat on the other side. This gentle spine stretch helps improve mobility in the spine and reduces the risk of vertebral fractures.

2. **Chest Opener Stretch**: Stand tall with your feet hip-width apart and your arms extended out to the sides at shoulder height. Gently squeeze your shoulder blades together as you bring your arms behind you, opening up the chest and stretching the muscles of the upper back. Hold the stretch for 15-30 seconds, then release. This chest opener stretch helps improve posture and reduce the risk of kyphosis (rounded upper back), a common complication of osteoporosis.

3. **Hamstring Stretch**: Sit on the edge of a chair with one leg extended straight in front of you and the other foot flat on the ground. Lean forward from the hips, reaching towards your toes with both hands. Keep your back straight and avoid rounding the spine. Hold the stretch for 15-30 seconds, then switch legs. This hamstring stretch helps improve flexibility in the back of the thighs and lower back, reducing the risk of falls and fractures.

4. **Wall Angel Stretch**: Stand with your back against a wall and your feet hip-width apart. Place your arms against the wall at shoulder height with your elbows bent to 90 degrees and your palms facing forward. Slowly slide your arms up the wall as high as you can while keeping your elbows and wrists in contact with the wall. Hold the stretch for 15-30 seconds, then lower your arms back down. This wall angel stretch helps improve shoulder mobility and strengthen the muscles of the upper back, reducing the risk of shoulder fractures.

Diabetes and Blood Circulation

Diabetes is a chronic condition characterized by high blood sugar levels, which can lead to various complications, including poor circulation. Reduced blood flow to the extremities can result in numbness, tingling, and increased risk of foot ulcers and infections.

Consider the following stretching exercises tailored for individuals managing diabetes:

1. **Calf Stretch**: Stand facing a wall with your hands resting against it at shoulder height. Step one foot back and press your heel into the ground, keeping your back leg straight and your knee bent. Feel the stretch in your back leg's calf as you slant slightly forward. Hold the stretch for 15-30 seconds, then switch legs. This calf stretch helps improve blood flow to the lower legs and feet, reducing the risk of cramps and improving mobility.

2. **Seated Toe Touch**: Sit on the ground with your legs extended in front of you and your feet flexed towards you. Engage your core and hinge forward at the hips, reaching towards your toes with your hands. Keep your back straight and avoid

rounding the spine. Hold the stretch for 15-30 seconds, then release. This seated toe touch stretch helps improve circulation in the legs and feet, reducing the risk of numbness and tingling.

3. **Ankle Circles**: Sit on a chair with your feet flat on the ground. Lift one foot off the ground and gently rotate your ankle in a circular motion, moving clockwise and counterclockwise to improve mobility and circulation. Repeat for 10-15 repetitions, then switch feet. This ankle circle exercise helps improve blood flow to the ankles and feet, reducing the risk of swelling and improving range of motion.

4. **Butterfly Stretch**: Sit on the ground with the soles of your feet together and your knees bent out to the sides. Hold onto your feet with your hands and gently press your knees towards the ground, feeling a stretch in the inner thighs and groin. Hold the stretch for 15-30 seconds, then release. This butterfly stretch helps improve circulation in the hips and lower body, reducing the risk of stiffness and discomfort.

Managing Chronic Pain through Stretching

Chronic pain is a complex condition that affects millions of individuals worldwide, impacting their quality of life and daily functioning. While medication and other treatments may provide temporary relief, stretching exercises offer a natural and holistic approach to managing chronic pain.

Consider the following stretching exercises tailored for individuals managing chronic pain:

1. **Cat-Cow Stretch**: Begin by placing your hands directly beneath your shoulders and your knees beneath your hips in the hands and knees position. Inhale as you arch your back, lifting your chest and tailbone towards the ceiling (Cow Pose). Exhale as you round your back, tucking your chin towards your chest and pressing into the ground with your hands (Cat Pose). Repeat for 5-10 repetitions, flowing smoothly between the two poses to release tension in the spine.

2. **Child's Pose:** Begin on your hands and knees with your toes touching and knees

apart. Sit back onto your heels and extend your arms forward, lowering your chest towards the ground and resting your forehead on the mat. Hold for 30-60 seconds, breathing deeply and allowing your entire body to relax and release tension.

3. **Standing Forward Fold:** Stand tall with your feet hip-width apart and your arms by your sides. Inhale as you reach your arms overhead, lengthening your spine and lifting your chest towards the sky. Exhale as you hinge forward at the hips, folding your torso over your legs and reaching towards the ground with your hands. Allow your head and neck to relax, feeling a stretch in the hamstrings and lower back. Hold for 15-30 seconds, then slowly roll up to standing.

4. **Seated Spinal Twist:** Take a seat on the floor and extend your legs in front of you. Bend one knee and cross it over the opposite leg, placing the foot flat on the ground. Place the opposite hand on the outside of the bent knee and

gently twist towards the bent leg, placing the other hand behind you for support. Hold for 15-30 seconds, then switch sides. This seated spinal twist helps release tension in the spine and reduce discomfort in the lower back and hips.

CHAPTER TEN:

Advanced Stretching Techniques

As individuals progress in their flexibility journey, they may seek out advanced stretching techniques to further enhance their range of motion, improve muscle strength, and optimize overall physical function.

Advanced stretching techniques go beyond basic static stretches and incorporate methods such as proprioceptive neuromuscular facilitation (PNF), yoga and Pilates, and the use of resistance bands and props.

In this section, we explore these advanced techniques and how they can benefit individuals looking to take their stretching routine to the next level.

Proprioceptive Neuromuscular Facilitation (PNF)

Proprioceptive neuromuscular facilitation, or PNF, is a stretching technique that involves a combination of passive stretching and muscle contraction to improve flexibility and enhance muscle strength.

PNF stretching utilizes the body's proprioceptors, which are sensory receptors located in the muscles and tendons, to facilitate a deeper stretch and increase range of motion.

There are several variations of PNF stretching, including the hold-relax technique, contract-relax technique, and contract-relax-antagonist-contract technique. Consider the following steps for performing a PNF stretch:

1. **Passive Stretch**: Begin by assuming a passive stretch position for the target muscle group. Hold the stretch for 10-15 seconds to lengthen the muscle and prepare it for the PNF technique.

2. **Isometric Contraction:** Next, engage the target muscle by contracting it

isometrically (without changing its length) against resistance for 5-10 seconds. Apply gentle pressure with your hand or a partner to resist the muscle contraction and increase the intensity of the stretch.

3. **Relaxation**: After the isometric contraction, relax the muscle completely and exhale deeply, allowing it to lengthen further as you deepen the stretch. Hold the relaxed stretch for 10-15 seconds.

4. **Repeat**: Repeat the cycle of contraction and relaxation 2-3 times, gradually increasing the intensity of the stretch with each repetition. Focus on maintaining smooth, controlled movements and avoiding any sudden or jerky motions.

Yoga and Pilates for Seniors

Yoga and Pilates are two popular mind-body practices that offer a holistic approach to improving flexibility, strength, and balance. Both disciplines incorporate a series of poses or exercises that target different muscle groups and movement patterns, promoting physical and mental well-being.

Consider the following key principles of yoga and Pilates for seniors:

1. **Gentle Movements**: Yoga and Pilates for seniors typically emphasize gentle, low-impact movements that are suitable for individuals of all fitness levels and abilities. Poses and exercises can be modified to accommodate physical limitations or health concerns, making them accessible to everyone.

2. **Breath Awareness**: Both yoga and Pilates place a strong emphasis on breath awareness, with practitioners encouraged to synchronize movement with the breath. Deep, diaphragmatic breathing helps reduce stress, promote relaxation, and improve oxygenation to the muscles and tissues.

3. **Mindfulness**: Yoga and Pilates encourage mindfulness and present-moment awareness, allowing seniors to focus their attention inward and cultivate a sense of calm and tranquility. Mindfulness practices can help reduce anxiety, improve mood, and enhance overall mental well-being.

4. **Balance and Stability**: Many yoga and Pilates poses involve balancing on one leg or maintaining stability in challenging positions, helping seniors improve balance, coordination, and proprioception. Stronger balance and stability can reduce the risk of falls and injuries, particularly in older adults.

5. **Flexibility and Strength**: Yoga and Pilates exercises are designed to improve flexibility, mobility, and muscle strength throughout the body. Regular practice can help seniors maintain or improve range of motion in the joints, reduce muscle stiffness, and enhance overall physical function.

Incorporating Resistance Bands and Props

Resistance bands and props are versatile tools that can enhance the effectiveness of stretching exercises and provide added resistance for building strength and stability. Consider the following ways to incorporate resistance bands and props into your stretching routine:

1. **Band-Assisted Stretching**: Use resistance bands to assist with passive stretching exercises, such as hamstring stretches or shoulder stretches. Anchor one end of the band to a stable object and loop the other end around the foot or hand of the target limb. Gently pull on the band to increase the intensity of the stretch and hold for 15-30 seconds.

2. **Band Resistance Exercises:** Perform resistance exercises using resistance bands to strengthen the muscles surrounding the joints and improve stability. Exercises such as bicep curls, shoulder presses, and leg lifts can be performed with resistance bands to target specific muscle groups and build strength.

3. **Foam Rollers and Massage Balls**: Incorporate foam rollers and massage balls into your stretching routine to release tension in the muscles and fascia. Roll over tight or sore areas of the body, applying gentle pressure to promote relaxation and reduce muscle stiffness. Use foam rollers and massage balls before or after stretching to improve flexibility and enhance recovery.

4. **Pilates Props:** Pilates props such as stability balls, resistance rings, and foam blocks can be used to add variety and challenge to your stretching routine. Perform exercises such as bridge lifts, leg circles, and spinal twists using Pilates props to target different muscle groups and improve overall body awareness and control.

CHAPTER ELEVEN:

Stretching for Daily Activities

In this section, we explore three key aspects of stretching for daily activities: stretching at home, stretching at work or while traveling, and integrating stretching into daily routines.

Stretching at Home

Home is often the most convenient and comfortable environment for incorporating stretching into your daily routine. With minimal equipment and space required, you can easily set aside time each day to focus on improving flexibility and mobility.

Consider the following tips for stretching at home:

1. **Designated Stretching Area**: Create a designated stretching area in your home where you feel comfortable and motivated to practice. This could be a corner of a room with a yoga mat or a clear space on the living room floor.

2. **Morning Routine**: Start your day off on the right foot by incorporating stretching into your morning routine. Spend 10-15 minutes performing a series of gentle stretches to wake up your muscles, improve circulation, and prepare your body for the day ahead.

3. **Evening Wind-Down**: Wind down in the evening with a relaxing stretching session to release tension from the day and promote relaxation before bedtime. Focus on gentle, soothing stretches to help calm the mind and prepare for restful sleep.

4. **Family Stretch Time**: Get the whole family involved in stretching by incorporating it into your daily routine. Set aside time each day for a family stretching session, where everyone can participate and reap the benefits of improved flexibility and mobility together.

5. **Variety of Stretches**: Mix up your stretching routine by incorporating a variety of stretches targeting different

muscle groups and movement patterns. This helps prevent boredom and ensures that you are addressing all areas of your body that may be tight or stiff.

Stretching at Work or While Traveling

Finding time to stretch while at work or while traveling can be challenging, but it's essential for maintaining physical comfort and preventing stiffness and fatigue. Consider the following tips for stretching at work or while traveling:

1. **Desk Stretches**: Take regular breaks throughout the workday to stretch at your desk. Perform simple stretches such as neck rolls, shoulder shrugs, and seated hamstring stretches to relieve tension and improve circulation.

2. **Micro-Breaks**: Incorporate short stretching breaks into your work routine by setting a timer to remind yourself to stretch every hour or so. Spend a few minutes performing quick stretches to counteract the effects of prolonged sitting and reduce muscle stiffness.

3. **Standing Desk**: If possible, use a standing desk or adjustable workstation to alternate between sitting and standing throughout the day. Take advantage of standing breaks to perform standing stretches such as calf raises, hip flexor stretches, and chest openers.

4. **Travel-Friendly Stretches:** While traveling, take advantage of downtime during layovers or long flights to stretch and move your body. Perform seated stretches, leg lifts, and shoulder rolls to improve circulation, reduce stiffness, and alleviate discomfort from prolonged sitting.

5. **Hotel Room Workouts**: If staying in a hotel, use your room as a makeshift workout space to perform stretching exercises and bodyweight movements. Follow along with online stretching videos or smartphone apps for guided stretching routines tailored to travelers.

Integrating Stretching into Daily Routines

Integrating stretching into your daily routines is key to making it a consistent and sustainable habit. Consider the following strategies for integrating stretching into your daily routines:

1. **Morning Ritual**: Start each morning with a few minutes of stretching as part of your morning ritual. Incorporate stretches into activities such as brushing your teeth, making coffee, or checking emails to kickstart your day with a burst of energy and vitality.

2. **Activity Transitions**: Use transitions between activities throughout the day as opportunities to stretch and move your body. Pause for a few moments between tasks to perform quick stretches, reset your posture, and refresh your mind.

3. **Routine Reminders**: Set reminders or cues throughout your day to prompt you to stretch. Use visual cues such as sticky notes or phone alerts to remind yourself to take stretching breaks at regular intervals.

4. **Multitasking Stretching**: Combine stretching with other activities you enjoy, such as watching TV, listening to music, or talking on the phone. Perform gentle stretches while engaging in these activities to maximize your time and incorporate stretching seamlessly into your day.

5. **Bedtime Stretch Routine**: Wind down in the evening with a bedtime stretch routine to relax your body and prepare for sleep. Spend 10-15 minutes performing gentle stretches to release tension from the day and promote restful sleep.

CHAPTER TWELVE:

Staying Motivated and Consistent

In this section, we explore three essential aspects of staying motivated and consistent: setting long-term goals, tracking progress and celebrating milestones, and finding support and accountability.

Setting Long-Term Goals

Setting long-term goals provides a clear direction and purpose for your stretching routine, helping you stay focused and motivated over time. When setting long-term goals for your stretching practice, consider the following factors:

1. **Specificity**: Make your goals as specific as possible, clearly defining what you want to achieve and why it's important to you. Instead of vague goals like "improve flexibility," set specific goals such as "touching toes without discomfort" or "achieving a full split."

2. **Measurability**: Ensure that your goals are measurable so that you can track your progress and assess your success. Use quantifiable metrics such as inches gained in flexibility, increased range of motion, or improved performance in specific activities.

3. **Achievability**: Set goals that are realistic and achievable within a reasonable timeframe. Consider your current level of flexibility, physical abilities, and lifestyle constraints when setting goals to ensure they are attainable.

4. **Relevance**: Align your goals with your personal values, interests, and motivations to increase their relevance and significance. Choose goals that resonate with you and inspire you to stay committed to your stretching routine.

5. **Time-Bound**: Set deadlines or target dates for achieving your goals to create a sense of urgency and accountability. Break down long-term goals into smaller, manageable milestones with specific timelines for completion.

Tracking Progress and Celebrating Milestones

Tracking your progress and celebrating milestones along the way is essential for maintaining motivation and momentum in your stretching journey. Consider the following strategies for tracking progress and celebrating milestones:

1. **Keep a Stretching Journal**: Maintain a stretching journal or logbook to record your daily stretching sessions, including the duration, intensity, and types of stretches performed. Use your journal to track changes in flexibility, range of motion, and overall physical comfort over time.

2. **Take Measurements**: Use measuring tools such as a tape measure or goniometer to track changes in flexibility and range of motion in specific muscle groups or joints. Take measurements regularly and compare them to baseline measurements to assess progress.

3. **Set Milestones**: Break down your long-term goals into smaller, achievable

milestones or benchmarks. Celebrate each milestone reached, whether it's touching your toes for the first time, achieving a deeper stretch in a particular pose, or mastering a new stretching technique.

4. **Visual Progress**: Take photos or videos of yourself performing stretching exercises at regular intervals to visually track your progress over time. Compare photos side by side to see visible improvements in flexibility, posture, and overall physical appearance.

5. **Reward Yourself**: Celebrate your achievements and milestones with rewards that reinforce your progress and motivate you to continue stretching. Treat yourself to a massage, a new workout outfit, or a special indulgence as a reward for reaching your goals.

Finding Support and Accountability

Finding support and accountability from others can greatly enhance your motivation and consistency in maintaining a stretching routine. Whether it's through friends, family, or online communities, having a support system in place can provide encouragement, guidance, and accountability when you need it most.

Consider the following ways to find support and accountability in your stretching journey:

1. **Buddy System**: Partner up with a friend, family member, or workout buddy who shares similar goals and interests. Hold each other accountable by scheduling regular stretching sessions together, providing encouragement and motivation, and celebrating achievements together.

2. **Join a Class**: Enroll in a group stretching class or workshop led by a qualified instructor. Group classes provide structure, guidance, and camaraderie, making it easier to stay motivated and consistent in your stretching practice.

3. **Online Communities**: Join online forums, social media groups, or fitness communities dedicated to stretching and flexibility. Connect with like-minded individuals, share your progress and

challenges, and seek advice and support from fellow members.

4. **Coach or Mentor:** Work with a qualified coach, personal trainer, or stretching instructor who can provide personalized guidance, feedback, and accountability. A coach can help you set realistic goals, develop an effective stretching routine, and overcome obstacles along the way.

5. **Accountability Apps**: Use smartphone apps or online tools designed to track your stretching progress and provide reminders and accountability. Set reminders for stretching sessions, log your workouts, and receive virtual encouragement and support to stay on track.

CHAPTER THIRTEEN:

Conclusion

As you reach the conclusion of "Stretching Exercises For Seniors Over 50," I hope you feel empowered and inspired to embark on a journey of improved flexibility, mobility, and overall well-being.

Throughout this book, we have delved into the importance of stretching for seniors, exploring its myriad benefits and providing practical guidance for incorporating stretching into your daily life.

By understanding the significance of stretching and its positive impact on physical and mental health, you have taken the first step towards a healthier and more active lifestyle.

From gentle warm-up exercises to targeted stretches for specific health conditions, you now possess a comprehensive toolkit to enhance your flexibility and mobility at any age.

Remember, consistency is key on this journey. Setting long-term goals, tracking your progress, and finding support and accountability will help you stay motivated and committed to your stretching routine.

Whether you're stretching at home, at work, or while traveling, every effort you make contributes to your overall health and well-being.

As you continue your stretching practice, listen to your body, honor its limitations, and celebrate its victories. Embrace the journey, savor the progress, and enjoy the transformative benefits of increased flexibility, reduced pain, and enhanced quality of life.

Thank you for investing your time and energy into improving your health and vitality through stretching. May this book serve as a valuable resource and companion on your path to optimal wellness.

Here's to a future filled with strength, mobility, and vitality—all achieved through the simple yet profound act of stretching.